SIMPLE GUIDE FOR KETO DIET

By : M.D.DEBWA

ISBN: 979-8-6374-1270-9

CONTENTS

INTRODUCTION

keto diet, is a diet often used to lose weight and treat some diseases. It is a high-fat, medium-protein, low-carbohydrate (starch and sugary) system. Mostly, 70% of your calories are from fat, 25% from protein and 5% from carbohydrates. I will explain in detail about the keto macros and how to calculate them. Also known as ketogenic dieting or ketogenic diet, it is classified in the scientific community as a low-carb or high-fat dieter.

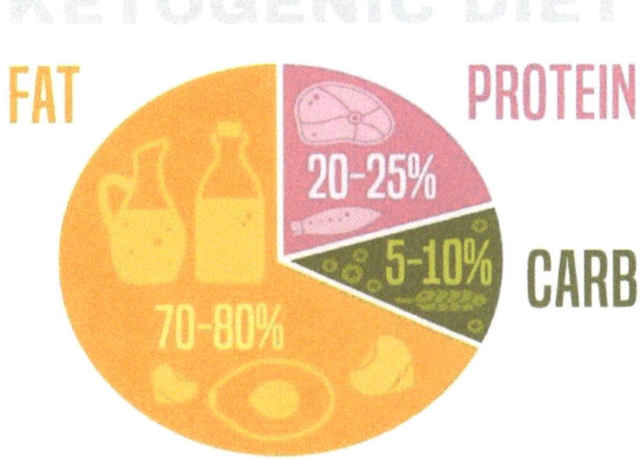

The idea of the keto diet is to minimize carbohydrates to a maximum (less than 20 to 50 grams of carbohydrates per day), and thus the body relies on fat (from food and from the body) as a source of energy instead of glucose, as it is rumored that low insulin levels in the body stimulate fat burning (Insulin is a hormone secreted by the pancreas to deal with glucose in the blood and transports it to cells to provide energy).

It should also be noted that the keto diet is not high in protein (Atkins Diet is high in protein, fat and low in carb), because high protein is converted to glucose by the process of Glucononeogenisis and reduces the manufacture of ketones in the liver. In this book I will explain to you the amount of protein required during the keto diet, because there is a common mistake in Arabic books, where they describe large amounts of protein.

The brain relies mainly on glucose for energy. When carbohydrates are severely cut, your liver begins to break down fats and convert them into Ketons in the liver. These ketones are transported in the blood and nourish the brain and the rest of the cells (since the fatty acids are not transmitted to the brain because of the blood barrier), and your body is then in the state of Ketosis.

Keto diet followers measure ketones in their blood or urine to ensure they are in the ketosis state. The level of ketones in the blood at the time is higher than 0.5mmol / L and ideally from 1.5 to 3 mmol / L, higher than that your body is in a dangerous condition called Ketoacidosis or ketoacidosis, I will talk about it later in the keto damage section.

It should be noted that measuring the amount of ketones in your blood is unnecessary, as the keto followers depend on an easier method which is to follow the side effects of the keto diet, such as increased urination, dryness of the throat, mouth and sweat changing. It should be noted that fasting also prolonged periods increases ketones in the blood (thus epilepsy was treated in the past). Since you cannot fast throughout life, the keto diet is used to achieve ketosis instead of fasting

What drives people to measure ketones in their blood or urine is the rumors of the benefits of staying in the state of ketosis for long periods. If you search on Google for ketogenic diet in foreign sites, you will find that the first search page in Google is sites that sell Quito systems, and you find on the Arab sites a lot of words without any scientific evidence or evidence, and even advise to eat open amounts of fruit and grains! So what is the truth about keto diet, its effectiveness for slimming, diabetes treatment, epilepsy, increasing athletic activity, concentration, reducing cholesterol, treating pimples, ovarian cyst, blood pressure, etc.? How to apply keto and how much do you slim it?

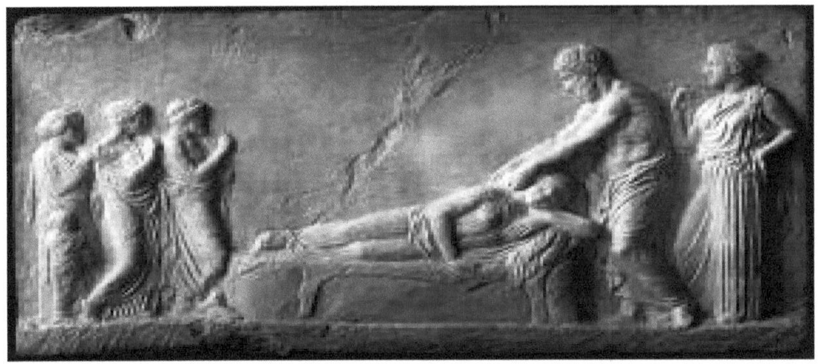

1 HISTORY OF THE KETO DIET

In ancient Greek medicine, they used to treat epilepsy by fasting for long periods of time, as a 500-BC biblical medical book appeared to a doctor about epilepsy. (Source).

The first modern scientific experiment to treat epilepsy with fasting was by French doctors in 1911 Guelpa & Marie, where doctors placed 20 people on a low-calorie vegetable diet with long periods of fasting. Doctors have already managed to treat two people, but the other 18 have failed to stick to this severe diet.

In 1921, American physician Rollin Woodyat discovered that the liver secreted beta-hydroxybutyrate, aceto-acetate, and acetone in the liver when following a low-carb, high-fat diet. These substances are called ketones.

Doctor Wilder of the Mayo Clinic built on this research and discovered ketones in the blood and called the diet "ketogenic diet", and used it successfully to treat epilepsy (especially in children), and said it is an alternative to fasting that is difficult to adhere to for long periods.

Dr. Woodyat's colleague, Mini Peterman, is the first to put macros for diet, 1 gram of protein per kg of weight, 10-15 grams of carbohydrates and the rest of calories from fat. Studies continued on the benefits and harms of keto and its side effects.

With the discovery of epilepsy drugs in 1938 (Dilantin), there was less interest in keto studies for treating epilepsy, but research on keto diet, its effectiveness for slimming, and its effectiveness to treat several diseases has continued to this day.

It is not yet known why fasting and keto epilepsy are treated. Is it because of ketones in the blood? Or because of a lack of glucose? Or because of a change in the salts of the body? The main effect of keto in the treatment of epilepsy is still mysterious

Summary of the history of keto: The topic started with the treatment of epilepsy with fasting by the ancient Greeks, then Western doctors experimented with fasting in the early twentieth century and found adherence to it difficult, so they moved to use the keto diet to treat epilepsy. Research continued on Keto to this day

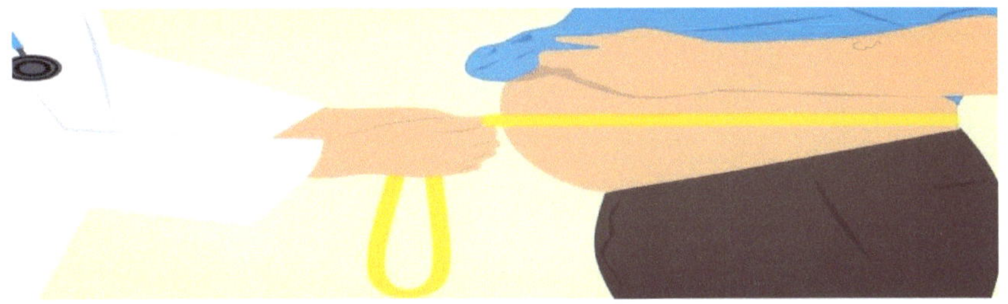

2 HOW DO YOU LOSE YOUR FAT ON IT?

There is a common mistake in many books, they say that you can eat open amounts of protein and fat and lose your weight as long as you block the carp! This is a mistake for a simple reason, which is that a lot of athletes and bodybuilders follow the dietary keto diet, that is, they eat large amounts of food to increase their weight, or even athletes follow it while maintaining their weight, and therefore your loss of fat depends mainly on the amount of food or calories you eat . If you suffer from weight loss during the keto diet, this is because you eat more food than required. Do not believe Arabic sites that advise you to eat open food with this diet.

Yes, there are some who do not weigh their food or count their calories and lose their fat on ketogenic diet, these people most of whom are obese. Once you cut carbohydrates, sugars, sweets, pastries, rice and pasta, a noticeable reduction in calories occurs due to reduced food options, and protein, fats and vegetables help a lot in satiety, so the fat person automatically eats less food than he used to eat.

However, people who are small in size or who are not obese may not succeed with them, as these people have a low calorie requirement (their metabolic rate is relatively low due to their small size), and therefore they need to control the quantities of food and calories more precisely in order to lose their weight at a good and continuous rate.

Fat loss occurs when you eat fewer calories than you consume daily. Your body consumes energy throughout the day for walking, movement, standing, sitting, homework, driving, and vital body functions such as breathing, taking out, digesting, and controlling body temperature and blood circulation ... etc.

This energy that you consume daily is called TDEE, Total Daily Energy Expenditure, or your daily caloric needs. This energy is measured in calories. Calorie: The amount of energy needed to raise a temperature of 1 kg of water 1 ° C.

So, in order to lose your weight on the ketogenic diet, or on any diet, you must calculate your daily caloric needs, and then consume an amount of calories less than 20% to 40%. Your body compensates for this caloric deficiency by burning your body fat.

Or, you can simply calculate your daily caloric needs with a simple formula: multiplying your weight in kilograms * 30
If your weight is 83 kg, your needs are calories = 83 * 30 = 2500 calories.
If you deduct 20% of the 2500, you eat 2000 calories a day, you create a 500-calorie deficit, and there is a weekly deficit = 7 * 500 = 3500 calories.
Since 1 kg of fat has about 7,000 calories, your body compensates for the 3,500-week deficit by burning half a kilogram of fat from your body.
If you eat 1500 calories a day, you create a deficit of 1,000 calories per day, that is, you create a deficit of 7000 calories per week and you lose 1 kg of your body fat per week.
You can, of course, increase your weight loss rate with iron exercises and increase non-athletic movement.

`If you are still a beginner and see calculating calories as a complicated matter for you, I later set out in this book tables for a ketogenic diet that you can walk on without calculation..

Summary How to lose weight on a keto diet: In order to lose weight on any diet, you must eat fewer calories than you consume. These are the simplest rules of thermodynamics, energy is neither fatal nor created. If you eat a large amount of fats, pans, and nuts, your weight may be proven. Do not believe sites that advise you to eat open amounts of food because they choose the easiest way to promote a product .

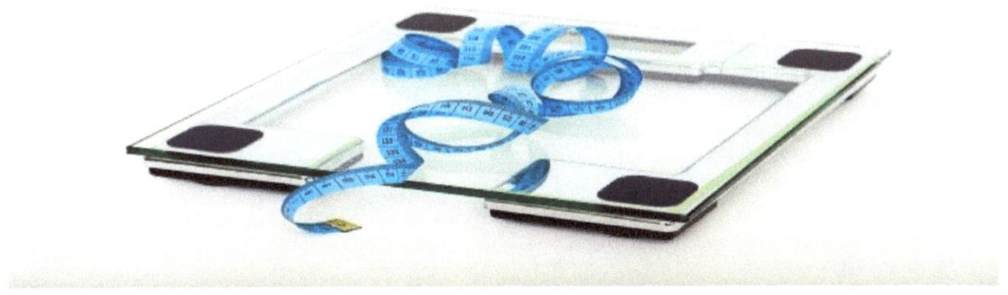

3 HOW TO START A KETO DIET ?

I got to know in a simple way what is Keto Diet (there is still a detailed explanation to come), and I got to know its history and how to lose weight on it. So how do you start?

There is an example that says, "Failure to plan is planning to fail." Without a plan in which you know where you are, where you are going, when you arrive, what steps and how to measure your progress, you will not succeed. He who walks on a diet without a plan, like a wanderer in the desert without a compass (or GPS) does not know where he is, where he is going, and when he gets there . I facilitated the steps as possible .

The First Steps To Getting Started With Keto Diet

The very simple first step, which is registering your weight, you may record it on an Excel or Word file or download the "Monitor Your Weight" application on your mobile.

The Second Step

Then, set a goal for your ideal weight. Perhaps an easy way is the man's height in cm - 100. I mean, if your height is 170 you subtract 100 from it, your ideal weight is 70. For a woman, her ideal weight is her height in cm - 105. I mean, if your height is 160, your ideal weight is

160-105 = 55 kg. This method is suitable for beginners and beginners.

As for the professional, he can measure the percentage of fat in meters, and then set the goal of 10% for men or 20% for women .

If you are a man and you weigh 80 kg and your fat percentage is 25% and you want to reduce it to 10%, you are required to lose 15% of your weight, i.e. a 12 kg loss.

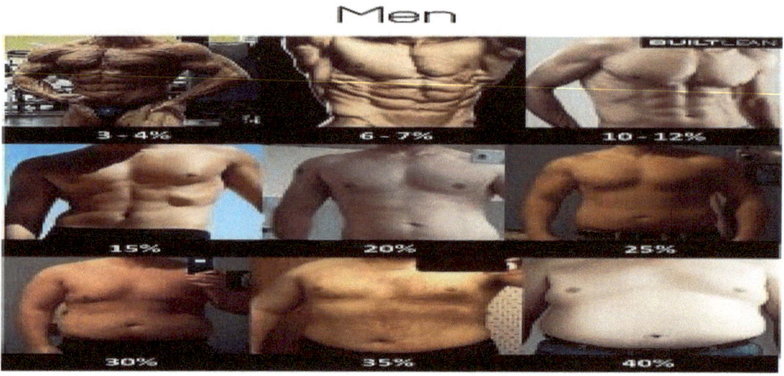

If you are a woman and you weigh 70 kg and your fat percentage is 35% and you want to reduce it to 20%, you are required to lose 15% of your weight, i.e. a loss of 10.5 kg. If you do not have a meter now, the first way is to discount 100 of your height with a poison to a man, or a 105-inch discount for a woman is sufficient

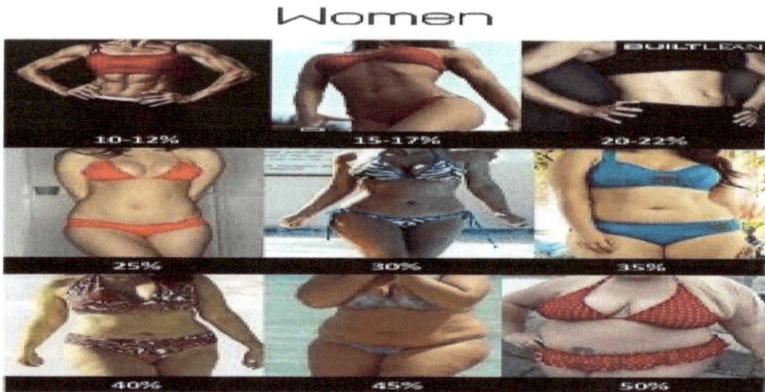

The Third Step

You now know how many kilograms you need to lose, a weekly weight loss rate required. A 1% weekly body weight is good for men and women of small sizes. If a man weighs 80 kg, an average loss of 0.8 kg is appropriate. If a woman weighs 70 kg, a loss rate of 0.7 kg is appropriate. People with large weights can lose 1.5% to 2% per week. I mean, if a man weighed 100 kg, his body would initially bear a loss of

1.5 to 2 kg per week. These are just nominations. You can select a suitable loss rate for your body, conditions and goal.

The Fourth Step

Determine the amount of calories you eat. Perhaps by deducting 20% or 40% of your caloric needs (your weight in kilograms * 30), this means that if you are a man and you weigh 90 kilograms, your caloric needs = 90 * 30 = 2700 calories. If you deduct 30% of them, you are required to deduct 810 calories, that is, you eat 1900 calories daily.

Or you can see the keto diet forms that I will write for you later and follow them as they are or change them according to your preference.

The Fifth Step

You will eat the amount of calories you set for a week, then measure your weight (or your weight + your fat percentage) again and record it (on the Excel file or the mobile app), and see whether you are achieving the required weekly weight loss rate or not.

If the required weekly loss rate is achieved, then well done, the amount of calories is set. If you achieve a slower rate than required, reduce your calories again from 100 to 200 calories, and your activity may increase slightly.

If you lose a large amount of weight (and muscles) and feel severe hunger and stress, then you eat a small amount of calories less than necessary and do not mind increasing them to ensure your continuity in the system and keep your muscles during the diet
The subject is very personal, every person has a calorie intake that suits them and it is very easy to take an experience and adjust your calories on your own.

The Last Step

It is cleaning your kitchen from sweets, pastries and sugars. This will make your commitment to the diet a lot easier. Buy a keto diet and fill your kitchen with it, and you may learn about keto recipes online because you will need them to ensure that it lasts for weeks and months. About this step, you must talk about what you can eat and what you cannot eat on the Keto Diet

Summary of "How to start the keto diet": to set your goal, the required weekly weight loss rate, and the amount of calories you are supposed to eat, then you follow your progress weekly and adjust your calories as needed. If you do not want the calculations, you can follow the Atkins diet.

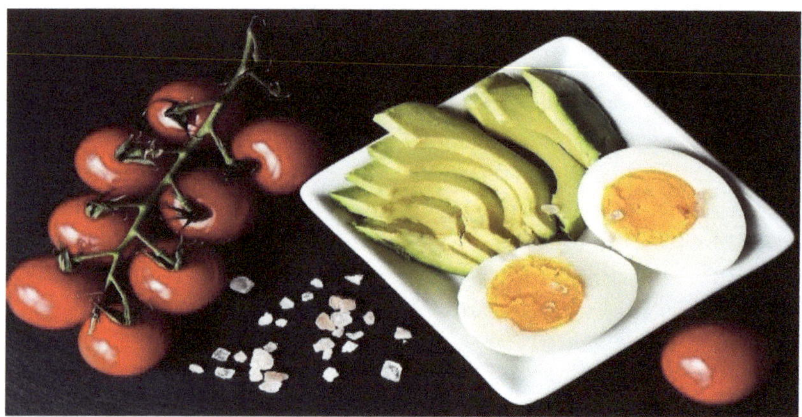

4 KETO DIET TABLE TO EAT

Here comes the talk about Macro Diet Keto. Macros are the nutrients for protein, carbohydrates and fats.
- 1 gram of protein = 4 calories
- 1 gram carb = 4 calories
- 1 gram of fat = 9 calories
- 1 to 1.6 grams of protein is required for your weight per kilogram of weight. The lowest number for a non-athlete and a higher number for an athlete

Less than 50 grams of carb (less than 20 grams puts you in a faster ketosis condition)
- The rest of the calories are from fat
- If you eat 2000 calories and weigh 80 kilograms, the macro is as follows :

1.6 * 80 = 128 grams protein
- That is 128 * 4 calories = 512 calories from protein
- 50 grams of carb * 4 calories = 200 calories of carbohydrates
- So, the remaining calories for fat are 2000 - 512 - 200 = 1288 calories
- Since each gram of fat has 9 calories, then 143 g of fat is required.

This is a sample diet diet (in grams)

Food	Quant (Gram)	Cals.	Protein	Carb.	Fat	Fibers
Meal 1						
Eggs Whole	200	294	25.16	1.54	19.88	0
Butter	20	143	0.17	0.01	16.22	0
Tomato	75	13.5	0.66	2.94	0.15	0
Cucumbers	100	15	0.65	3.63	0.11	0
Cheddar Cheese	100	403	24.90	1.28	33.14	0
Any Food Kind Adding +						
Total		868.9	51.54	9.40	69.50	1.40

Food	Quant (Gram)	Cals.	Protein	Carb.	Fat	Fibers
Meal 2						
Cooked Chicken Breast	150	247.5	45	0	6	0
Olive Oil	20	176.8	0	0	20	0
Zucchini	100	17	1.20	3.10	0.30	1
Mushroom	50	11	1.54	1.64	0.17	0.50
Onion	50	20	0.55	4.50	0.05	0.85
Carrots	50	20.50	0.47	4.79	0.12	1.40
Any Food Kind Adding +						
Total		492.8	48.76	14.03	26.64	3.75

Food	Quant (Gram)	Cals.	Protein	Carb.	Fat	Fibers
Meal 3						
Mixed nuts	40	246	6.20	6.80	22.48	2.20
Cucumbers	100	15	0.65	3.63	0.11	0
Watercress	75	8.25	1.73	0.97	0.07	0.38
Lettuce	100	14	0.90	2.97	0.14	1.20
FullCream Cheese	100	316	20	1.60	24.17	0
Any Food Kind Adding +						
Total		599.25	29.48	15.97	47.50	4.28

Quantity	Cals.	Protein	Carb.	Fat	Fibers
Total Of 1 Day	1960.95	129.78	39.40	143.64	9.43

Note that 150 grams of chicken does not mean 150 grams of protein. 150 grams chicken contains 45 grams of protein, 0 grams of carbohydrates and 6 grams of fat.

Note that carbohydrates are 39 grams, meaning less than the maximum 50 grams. For information, in keto we calculate the net carb, that is, "net carp", and net carp = total carp size - fibers = 39-9 = 30

I postponed this information to you, so as not to be distracted at first. This is because the fibers do not convert into glucose in the blood.

So, as I understood from the keto macros, we need protein foods and high-fat food, and we need to avoid high-carp foods (or net carp).

Keto Diet Cuisine

. Meat, poultry, fish (especially high-fat fish such as sardines, anchovies, and mackerel because they contain excellent amounts of omega-3)

. Sausage, sausage, luncheon, and chanting

. Eggs (boiled and fried)

• Whey protein supplement and casein protein, especially low-carb like ISO 100

. High-fat cheese "cheddar, mozzarella, feta, parmesan, colby, gouda and ricotta"

• Butter, natural ghee, olive oil, coconut oil, linseed oil (hot oil), sesame oil, walnut oil (preferably away from commercialized wasted oils)

• Full cream cream

• Sauce and high-fat dressing (mayonnaise, garlic sauce, avocado sauce, etc.) Check the sauce feed card and ensure that it is low in carp.

. Avocado

. Greek Yogurt low carb

. Calculated amounts of nuts (and butter nuts like peanut butter and almonds) to control net carp

. Vegetables, especially leafy: arugula, basil, pepper, garlic, onion, cucumber, parsley, broccoli, zucchini, cauliflower and radish. (For squash, carrots, tomatoes, onions and beets, eat calculated amounts)

. Meat, chicken and broth soup

. Salt, black pepper, chili, all kinds of spices, vinegar, soy sauce, mustard

• Tea, coffee, nescafe (without white sugar but you can add heavy cream or low carb bleach), diet cola

• Sugar diet.

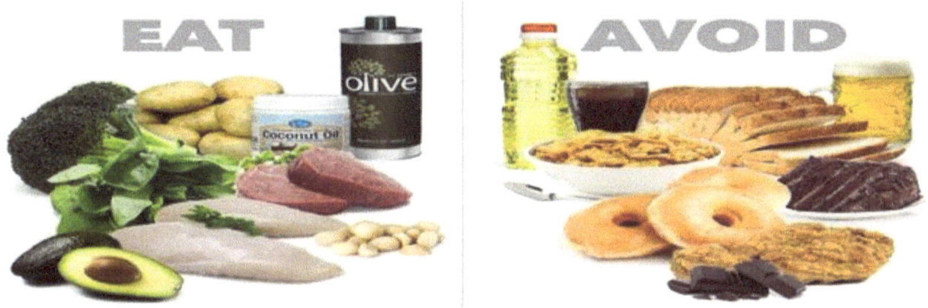

What You Don't Eat With Keto Diet ?

Pastries, baked goods, sweets, sugars•

. The fruit

• Sugar and white honey

. Starches (bread, pasta, fries, fries, and corn)

. Legumes (beans, lentils, chickpeas, lupine, white beans, red beans, beans)

. Grains (oats, bulgur, corn flakes, couscous, barley, wheat, and night)

• High-sugar soft drinks

. Milk is high in carp, and yogurt is skim too. Eat high-fat cheese better.

You can see a calorie table in the end of this book, which the amount of carbohydrates is written in all foods to know what to refrain from and what you are heading for . Or when you buy a product, see its nutrition card.

What About Dark Chocolate ?

Do not mind, provided that you calculate it in the net carp in your day and that it is 90% cocoa. The 70% cocoa is higher in sugar .

Summary "What you eat and not eat on the keto diet: to eat meat, cheese, vegetables and fats in calculated quantities and macros, and refrain from eating high carp foods as much as you can

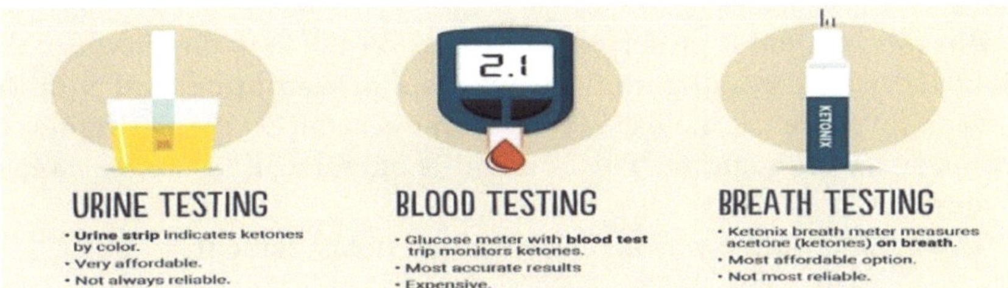

5 HOW DO YOU MEASURE KETONES IN YOUR BODY ?

I do not see the necessity to use techniques and devices to measure ketones in your body. You can count on following the side effects of keto :

• Increased urination: as the keto diet is a diuretic at first and you lose a large amount of water on it.

• Dry mouth and change its smell: the throat dries up due to a large loss of water, and the smell of yourself changes due to the escalation of acetone in the breath. The smell of acetone is like the smell of nail polish remover.

• Odor change in body or sweat: due to the rise of acetone in the sweat.

The common method is to use keto steaks or keto sticks and wink them in the urine. Depending on the color that appears on the lute, you know the amount of ketones and how much ketosis.

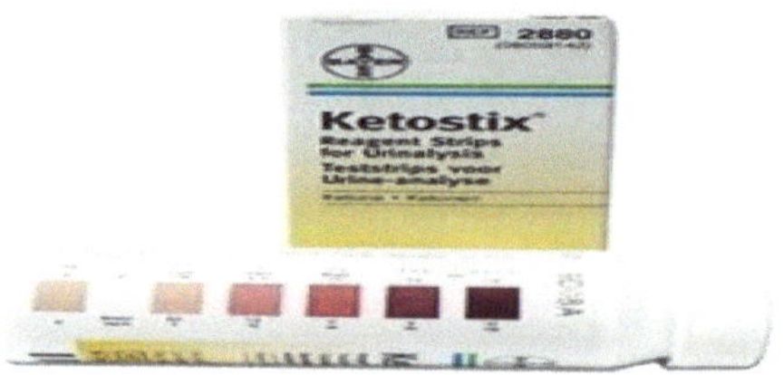

But this method is criticized by experts on the keto diet because the sticks measure the amount of Acetoacetate in your urine, and with the passage of time in ketosis, your kidney reduces the secretion of Acetoacetate in the urine. This method is only useful in the first weeks of your diet.

The most accurate way is to use a blood measurement

This device is sold in the range of $50 and is called the Keto meter, but a single analysis sheet costs $5, and therefore daily analysis is expensive. You may only do the analysis once or twice a week. To be in ketosis, the device should read from 0.5 to 3 mmol / L.

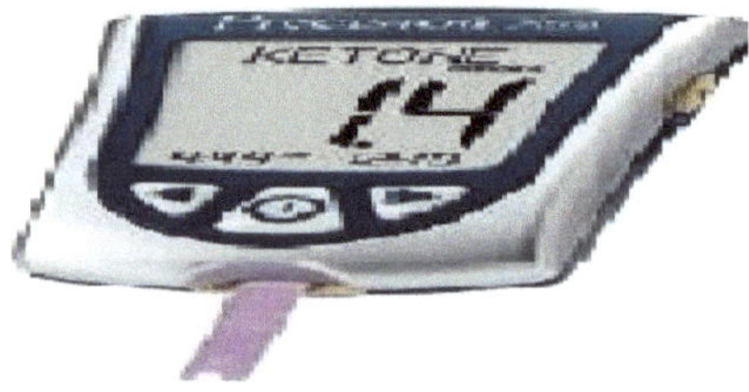

We should change how we contemplate the person. It seems as though we are permitting them to begin with a fresh start once more. You won't permit the circumstance to cause you or the gatherings required to hurt you anymore. This requires an elevated level of enthusiastic knowledge, discretion, and love. Absolution isn't simply "letting them free" for what they did, it is permitting those included to quit choosing not to move on and proceed onward to progressively significant things.

Summary of "How to measure ketones in your body": Measuring ketones is not necessary, you can follow the side effects of keto diet to make sure that you are in a ketosis condition, but if there is a reason that leads you to measure the extent of ketosis, I advise you to use a blood test by purchasing a device from Amazon and not urine sticks Keto Steaks .

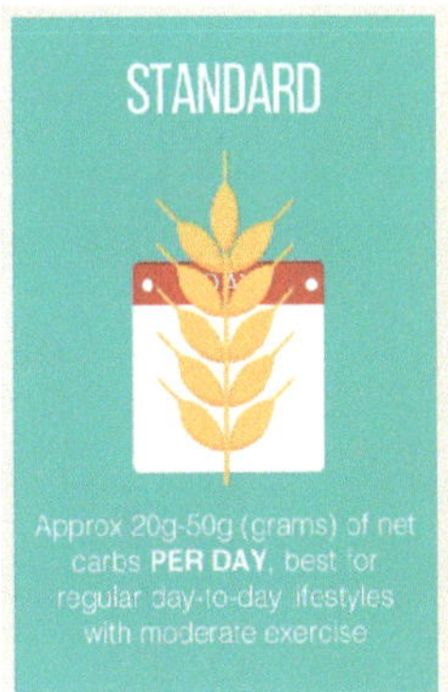

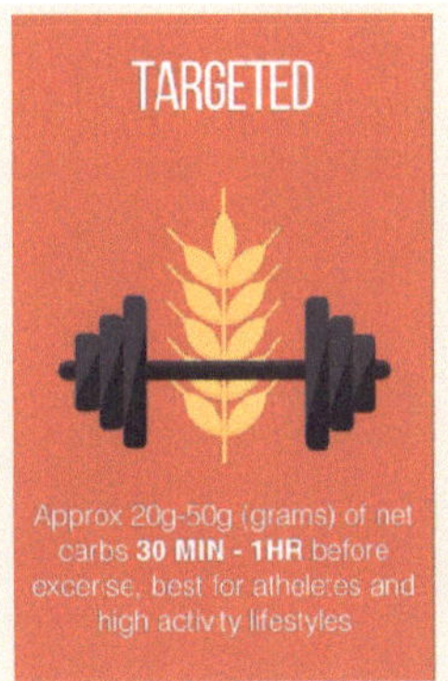

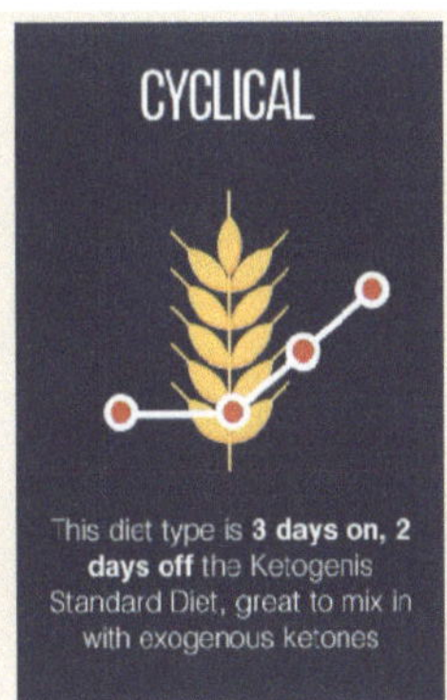

6 TYPES OF KETO DIET

This system in the book is Standard Keto Diet, SKD or the traditional keto diet. It relies on continuing as long as possible at the lowest net carb ratio (less than 50 grams) without Carb Refeeding. It is suitable for diabetic patient 2 or who has a medical condition that requires staying in ketosis as long as possible (such as epilepsy), or for beginners in general.

There are two other types, Cyclic Keto Diet CKD and Targeted Keto Diet TKD, in which you eat carp at certain times to refill glycogen stores in the muscles and liver.

- CKD: It is a low carb diet throughout the week, but at the end of the week you take a day of high carp and calories (400-600 grams carb) in order to refill the glycogen stores in your muscles. Suitable for bodybuilders and those who do light workouts throughout the week.

- TKD: It is a low-carb diet throughout the day, except for half an hour before exercise, as you eat 50 grams of absorbed carp. Suitable for those who play violent sports.

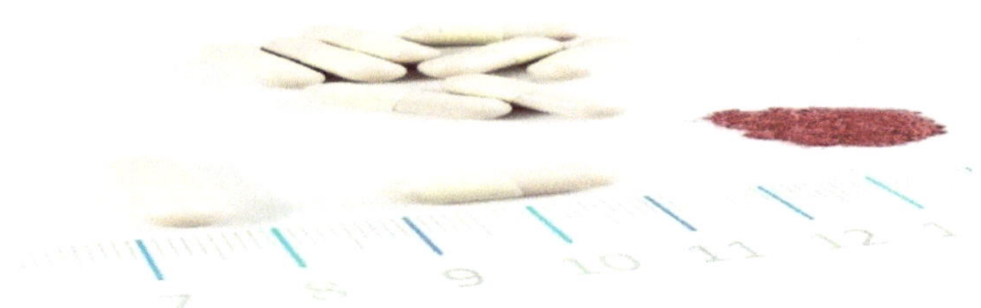

7 DIETARY SUPPLEMENTS DURING KETO

I discussed with you everything related to food during the keto, but with the carp pieces of starches, grains, fruits and legumes, you will need some supplements and salts not available in the keto foods, otherwise your health will be very tired and you lose your muscles and get out of the diet due to weakness and fatigue. These supplements are:

1- Multivitamin: to ensure that there is no deficiency of 13 vitamins and 9 minerals.

2- Fish Oil: This supplement is beneficial for anyone who does not eat fatty fish (sardines, mackerel, anchovies, or tuna) adequately.

3- Table salt: Contains sodium / potassium / iodine, like Dr. Salt

4- Magnesium supplement (400 mg in the evening): The main source of magnesium is whole grains, and you do not consume them.

5- Vitamin D supplement: The dosage of the supplement is according to the amount of your deficit, you should analyze.

6- Any other supplement that complements the deficiency in your diet program Additionally, putting yourself under this kind of pressure will leave you feeling dissatisfied in the end.

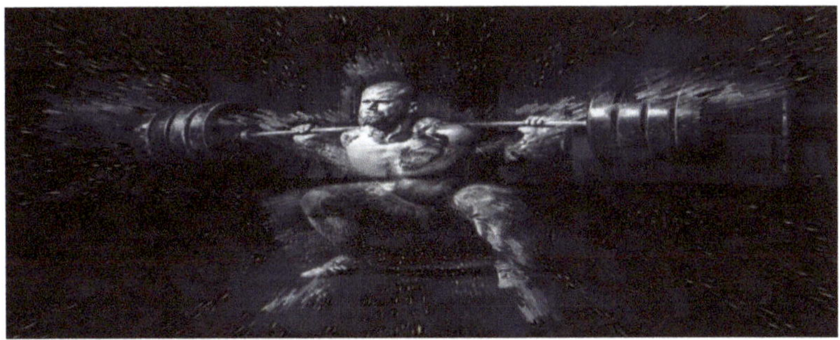

Benefits Of A ketogenic Diet

1 - Keto diet is effective in treating children with epilepsy, especially those who are resistant to epilepsy drugs. Because of this ancient benefit known for decades, scientists have tried keto to treat other cerebrovascular and neurological diseases such as Parkinson, Alzheimer's, multiple sclerosis, insomnia, autism and brain cancer. No study has found a benefit of keto for treating these diseases other than epilepsy .(Source : https://www.health.harvard.edu/blog/ketogenic-diet-is-the-ultimate-low-carb-diet-good-for-you-201707272712089)

2 - Of course, the ketogenic diet is effective for slimming, especially for people with insulin resistance and diabetes 2 or exposed to it. But what about healthy people? Is diet keto effective for dieting high carbohydrates ?

The answer is no. You can lose the same weight on a high-carb diet if you eat a high-protein diet. There are several studies that compared keto diet and high-carb diet with the same calories and the same amount of protein, and found the same result in weight loss after a long period (Study 1 : https://www.ncbi.nlm.nih.gov/pubmed/27903520) (Study 2 : http://www.cell.com/cell-metabolism/abstract/S1550-4131(15)00350-2) (Study3:http://ajcn.nutrition.org/content/early/2016/07/05/ajcn.116.133561.abstract). What makes Keto so special is that you lose a huge amount of water when you start with it.

3 - The benefit of ketogenic dieting compared to the high-carb dieting is more pronounced for people with diabetes 2 (source:https://www.ncbi.nlm.nih.gov/pubmed/15897479).

4- Keto diet increases satiety (source:https://sci-fit.net/ketogenic-diet-hunger-suppression/), but this is short-term. In the long run, sticking to it for many months may be difficult for many (but not all) people.

5 - There are common benefits between keto and any healthy diet that you lose weight with (with exercise of course). These benefits are not exclusive to Keto :

- Decreasing harmful cholesterol and beneficial cholesterol.

- Prevention of cancer and heart disease.

- Low blood pressure and triglycerides.

- Low insulin resistance and improved blood sugar levels.

- Increased male hormone.

- Treating depression, insomnia and stress.

- Feeling light.

6 - Treating acne or pills : There are new and emerging studies that have proven effective for keto diet on acne treatment (source:https://www.researchgate.net/publication/221825592_Nutrition_and_Acne_Therapeutic_Potential_of_Ketogenic_Diets).

7 - May help treat migraines (source:https://www.researchgate.net/blog/post/less-carbs-more-fat-ketogenic-diet-treats-migraine-patients) .

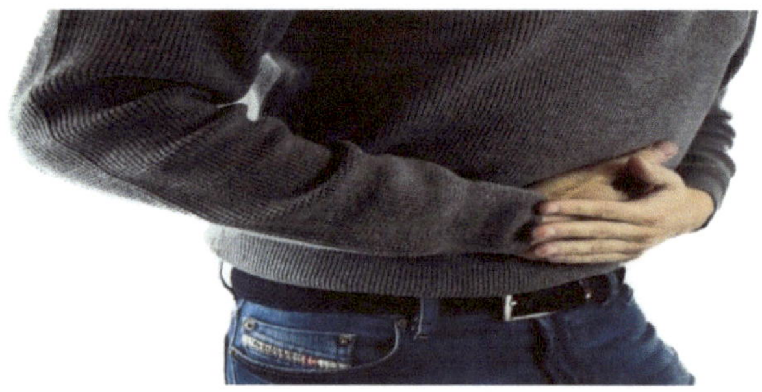

Ketogenic Diet Damages

Before mentioning harm to healthy people, it should be noted who should avoid dieting keto :
- People with kidney, liver and pancreas diseases.

- Diabetics 1 who take insulin, consult their physician and

continuously measure blood sugar levels and the level of ketosis in the blood to avoid ketoacidosis.

- Pregnant and lactating women.

- Children without medical supervision. Do not try the diet on your children.

- Executives or referrers must consult their physician first.

1 - The biggest harm is : No one knows the long-term harm of keto diet. Most studies that find benefits (or damages) to keto diet are done in a short period. Less than a year at best (source:https://www.health.harvard.edu/blog/ketogenic-diet-is-the-ultimate-low-carb-diet-good-for-you-2017072712089). So what does this mean to you ?
Either follow this diet with a doctor, or nutritionist, or educate yourself a lot before starting it, with periodic analyzes every 3 or 6 months, such as cholesterol, triglycerides, vitamin D, kidney and liver functions, and cumulative sugar, and possibly a complete blood picture. This diet is not 100% guaranteed in the long run, and you cannot believe who promotes this.

2- Many people eat more red meat, especially processed. And science has found that processed red meat increases the chance of several types of cancer .
(source:http://www.who.int/features/qa/cancer-red-meat/en/). That is, you are required to rely more on white meat and fish, and reduce the processed red meat as much as you can.

3- What is Ketoacidosis ?
Do not confuse ketosis and ketoacidosis. With ketosis, the rate of ketones in your blood ranges from 0.5 mmol / L to 3 mmol / L.
Ketoacidosis occurs in people with type 1 diabetes in the absence of insulin injections (and patients with type 2 diabetes in some cases). Since glucose does not reach their cells due to the absence of insulin, the body begins to secrete a large amount of ketones in the blood, reaching more than 10 mmol / L. Common symptoms of ketoacidosis are :
- Vomiting
- Rapid breathing and shortness of breath.
- frequent urination.
- Colic.
- dehydration and intense thirst.

- High blood glucose (not with keto).

More on ketoacidosis .
(source:https://ar.wikipedia.org/wiki/%D8%AD%D9%85%D8%A7%D8%B6_%D9%83%D9%8A%D8%AA%D9%88%D9%86%D9%8A_%D8%B3%D9%83%D8%B1%D9%8A).

As long as you follow the keto diet as described in this book , there is no way for your ketoacidosis to occur.

4- Keto flu :
Keto flu is simply a symptom of carbohydrate withdrawal. When you cut carbs suddenly in the early days of keto, it affects you :

- Dizziness
- Nausea
- Diarrhea or constipation
- Headache
- Fatigue
- Cramp
- Nervousness

To avoid these symptoms, you can :

1- Reducing carbohydrates or calories gradually, not suddenly.

2- Drink enough water daily (make sure your urine is always light, not yellow).

3- Eat a sufficient amount of minerals and salts (see the supplement section) such as sodium, potassium and magnesium.

4- Like any diet, your food should be healthy. Eat lots of vegetables and fiber. You will not feel healthy on mostly Kentucky and Big Mac food without bread.

8 COMMON QUESTIONS

1 - How much is it lowered or thinner on keto ?

This is the most common question. The amount of weight that you can lose depends on the amount of calories you eat. If your needs are 2500 calories per day and you eat 2000 calories, you will create a shortfall of 500 calories per day, or 3500 calories per week and lose half a kilogram of fat (1 kilogram of fat with 7000 calories). If you ate 1500 calories, you would create a deficit of 1,000 calories and lose 1 kg per week. Sports, cardio, and non-athletic movement also play a role in the amount of weight you lose.

You can try an appropriate amount of calories and adjust according to your need to get off according to your ability to carry the diet. Personally, I prefer a quick landing

2 - Is the keto diet suitable for bodybuilding ?

Carbohydrates are the body's favorite energy in power and explosive exercises that consume a short period of high intensity. Thus, you will lose some strength and less weights in the gym. It might be better for you to follow the Cyclic Keto Diet or Targeted Keto Diet so that you refill glycogen stores in your muscles every period to keep your strength high.

And don't believe some professional bodybuilders who swear on a ketogenic diet because they take steroids and their strength is not affected by any diet. These people may sell a system and promote the keto without real support.

3 - Is it suitable for pregnant women ?

During pregnancy, there is no way you can lose weight (unless you are obese). During the first 3 months of pregnancy, your goal is to stabilize your weight by eating your caloric needs. From month 3 to 7, you need to increase 300 calories over your needs in order for your weight and weight to increase your fetus at a reasonable rate. The other two months you need to add an additional 500 calories.

Trying to lose weight while pregnant is an intentional killing of a fetus. How do you lose weight and increase the weight of the fetus at the same time? (Exceptionally, obese patients are excluded).

The keto is also the last recommended system for a pregnant woman. You cut cereals, fruit, legumes, starches and milk, and you may develop a nutritional deficiency. Pregnant women basically need to increase vitamins and minerals, so how do you put yourself in an additional deficit?

Keto also has side effects such as headache, fatigue, dizziness and dehydration. So does it make sense to add this to the side effects of pregnancy? Forget it completely, my dear sister, and do not think about losing your weight during pregnancy with any diet as long as you do not have dangerous obesity, or at least under close medical supervision to preserve the health of the fetus.

4 - How long is the keto diet ?

You can walk for months to reach your ideal weight. Like any diet, you must ensure that you eat all the nutrients, vitamins and minerals your body needs so that your health does not get tired after a while and you become food-deficient.

5 - What is the effect of diet sugar and cola diet on keto ?

Diet sugar and cola diet do not contain glucose or any sugar, do not affect insulin in the blood and do not get you out of the ketosis state. They are appropriate for Keto Diet, and whoever says otherwise does see his guide and make sure that his words are only his personal opinion.

6 - Can intermittent fasting and the keto diet be followed together ?

Yes, intermittent fasting is 16-hour fasting and eating in an 8-hour window. Meaning that if you wake up at 8 in the morning, you ignore breakfast and then eat your first meal for 2 pm, and your last meal is 10 pm (window of 8 hours from

2 to 10). You eat macros and your keto diet, then fast from 10 pm until 8 the next morning.

7 - What are the stages of the ketogenic diet ?

Some are confused, because the Atkins diet contains 4 stages. There are no so-called ketogenic phases. The matter is that some people get tired of suddenly reducing carbohydrates and suffer from stress, nausea, dehydration and headache, and therefore they can gradually reduce carbohydrates.

Week 1 : 100 grams carbohydrates.

Week 2 : 75 grams carbohydrates.

And then cut carbohydrates under 50 grams, meaning 3 stages if you like .

8 - What is the appropriate sport?

I highly recommend iron exercises with keto to maintain and even increase your muscle mass. Muscles are active tissues that consume calories throughout the day. The higher your muscle mass, the higher your rate of burning.

Iron exercises also have several benefits :

- Increased bone density

- Tightening the body, flabs and slimming the belly and buttocks

- Increase the strength of ligaments and tendons

- Improve psychological and treatment of stress and depression

- Protection from heart disease and cancer

9 ADDITIONAL TABLES

A- Standard Keto Diet Plan Shopping List :

Meats and eggs	✔ Free-range eggs ✔ Fish (salmon is best due to fat content) ✔ Bacon ✔ Beef ✔ Salami/sausage ✔ Pork ✔ Chicken/poultry ✔ Wild game
Vegetables and fruits	✔ Green leafy vegetables (spinach, kale, arugula, etc.) ✔ Mushrooms ✔ Blueberries ✔ Artichoke hearts . ✔ Tomatoes ✔ Avocado ✔ Cucumber ✔ Zucchini ✔ Fresh spices ✔ Strawberries ✔ Blackberries ✔ Raspberries ✔ Bok Choy ✔ Cabbage ✔ Radishes ✔ Lemons ✔ Limes ✔ Asparagus
Fats and oils	✔ Olive oil ✔ Coconut oil ✔ Avocado oil ✔ Butter ✔ Canola oil
Cheese and Dairy	✔ Soft cheeses (Brie, Camembert, Parmesan, etc.) ✔ Hard cheeses (cheddar, Colby, Swiss, etc.) ✔ .. Cream cheese ✔ String (mozzarella) cheese ✔ 4% fat cottage cheese ✔ Whole milk yogurt ✔ Sour cream ✔ Goat cheese
Spices and condiments	✔ All plain spices ✔ Mayonnaise
Nuts	✔ Macadamia nuts ✔ Almonds ✔ Brazil Nuts ✔ Walnuts ✔ Pine nuts ✔ Peanuts ✔ Unsweetened nut butters
Other	✔ Coconut cream ✔ Coffee ✔ Keto-approved flour ✔ Oat fiber ✔ Unsweetened non-dairy milk (almond, coconut, etc.)

B - Standard Keto Diet Two Weeks Plan :

Week 1

Monday

- Breakfast : Two-egg omelet with spinach and mushrooms cooked in coconut oil
- Snack : Handful of blueberries
- Lunch : Chicken salad with artichoke hearts + tomatoes + mixed greens + boiled egg + olive oil
- Dinner : Seared salmon and a mixed green salad with avocado and olive oil

Tuesday
- Breakfast : Two fried eggs in olive oil and 1/2 of avocado with tomato and cilantro salsa
- Snack : Soft cheese with cucumber slices
- Lunch : Bacon-Lettuce and Tomato (BLT) on cloud bread
- Dinner : Zoodles with ground beef and homemade tomato sauce

Wednesday
- Breakfast : Bacon and eggs cooked in bacon fat
- Snack : Handful of macadamia nuts
- Lunch : Roast beef, brie, arugula, pesto, and olive plate
- Dinner : Shrimp, tomato, and avocado salad with olive oil and lime

Thursday
- Breakfast : Frittata with broccoli
- Snack : Celery and peanut butter
- Lunch : Turkey slices + almonds + avocado + cucumber + blueberries
- Dinner : Lamb chops with herb butter

Friday
- Breakfast : Scrambled eggs in butter with tomato and cilantro
- Snack : Green peppers with cream cheese
- Lunch : Salami and mayo + string cheese + radishes + avocado and olive oil
- Dinner : Chicken salad on lettuce with tomato

Saturday
- Breakfast : Boiled eggs with mayonnaise
- Snack : Pork rinds
- Lunch : Chicken salad in a jar with greens of your choice + olive oil
- Dinner : Roasted chicken and cabbage with mayo

Sunday
- Breakfast : Eggplant hash (eggplant seared in olive oil) topped with fried eggs.
- Snack : Homemade zucchini chips
- Lunch : Salami + roasted pepper + mixed green salad
- Dinner : Baked salmon with pesto and Brussels sprouts

Week 2

Monday
- Breakfast : Huevos rancheros (fried egg with tomato salsa, avocado and sour cream on the side)
- Snack : Handful of strawberries
- Lunch : Pepperoni and cream cheese rolls + celery slices +cherry tomatoes + almonds
- Dinner : Beef in cream sauce and steamed zucchini

Tuesday
- Breakfast : Keto coconut porridge (coconut flour + egg + coconut oil + coconut cream mixed together over a saucepan - try this recipe) topped with raspberries
- Snack : Cheese
- Lunch : Bacon, avocado, and French onion dip sandwich on cloud bread with almonds and blueberries
- Dinner : Pan-fried pork

Wednesday
- Breakfast : Blackberry and strawberry smoothie with coconut milk and lemon juice
- Snack : Fresh ham & cheese roll-ups
- Lunch : 2 boiled eggs + string cheese + avocado slices + cucumber + cottage cheese for dipping
- Dinner : Cooked chicken meatballs with zoodles and parmesan cheese

Thursday
- Breakfast : Two fried eggs over kale sautéed in olive oil
- Snack : Butter melted into coffee

- <u>Lunch</u> : Tuna salad with mixed greens dressed with olive oil + handful of raspberries

- <u>Dinner</u> : Chicken stir-fry in canola oil with bok choy and cabbage

Friday
- <u>Breakfast</u> : Low-carb blueberry pancakes (eggs + cream cheese + butter + almond flour + oat fiber + lemon zest + baking powder + blueberries - or try this recipe)

- <u>Snack</u> : Celery and cream cheese

- <u>Lunch</u> : Sauteed chicken and broccoli, two pieces of Babybel cheese, celery, and cream dipping sauce

- <u>Dinner</u> : Bacon-wrapped asparagus and brie

Saturday
- <u>Breakfast</u> : Baked eggs with tomato and sausage

- <u>Snack</u> : Cucumber and mayo

- <u>Lunch</u> : Smoked salmon and avocado plate

- <u>Dinner</u> : Scallop avocado salad

Sunday
- <u>Breakfast</u> : Green smoothie (avocado + MCT oil + cucumber + spinach + parsley + hemp seeds + turmeric + lemon)

- <u>Snack</u> : Handful of Brazil nuts

- <u>Lunch</u> : Chicken salad sandwich with cloud bread + macadamia nuts + blackberries

- <u>Dinner</u> : Zucchini lasagna (ground beef + mozzarella + parmesan + zucchini slices)

Table Of Calories In Food

This table is reviewed periodically and the data is consistent with the website of the US Department of Agriculture.

Food Name	Qty	Cals.	Protein	Carb	Fats	Fibers
Beef (cooked ,stewed or broiled)	100 grams	250	25	0	13	0
Roast beef	100 grams	267	21.9	0	17.32	0
Beef ground packaged frozen	100 grams	202	18.3	5	12	0.4
Beef Ground 3% (cooked ,stewed or broiled)	100 grams	151	27	0	3	0
Beef Ground 10% (cooked ,stewed or broiled)	100 grams	214	27	0	10	0
Kofta	100 grams	271	26	0	18	0
Beef Shank Cooked	100 grams	201	33	0	6.4	0
"Veal leg top round boneless cooked grilled	100 grams	128	27	0	2.2	0

Food Name	Qty	Cals.	Protein	Carb	Fats	Fibers
Full rump cooked broiled	100 grams	168	33.7	0	2.7	0
Rib steaks	100 grams	354	23	0	29	0
Mortadella	100 grams	311	16	3	25	0
Hot Dog Raw	100 grams	289	10	4	26	0
Sausages beef cooked	100 grams	331	18	0	28	0
Beef franks smoked raw	100 grams	137	13	6.5	6.5	1
Meat smoked turkey breast	100 grams	109	17.4	2.2	3	0
Turkey Mortadella	100 grams	109	17.4	2.2	3	0
Chicken Breast Raw Without Skin	100 grams	110	23	0	1	0
Chicken Breast (cooked ,stewed or broiled)	100 grams	165	30	0	4	0
Squab Pigeon cooked	100 grams	141	21.8	0.3	5.1	
Frozen Chicken Burger Raw	100 grams	240	17	5.5	16	0

Food Name	Qty	Cals.	Protein	Carb	Fats	Fibers
Chicken breast breaded fried	100 grams	270	21.7	9.4	16.5	3
Chicken Broth , Soup	100 grams	16	2	0.5	0.6	0
Beef broth soup	100 grams	88	9	0	4	0
Chicken Leg (cooked ,stewed or broiled)	100 grams	212	23.68	0	12.28	0
Duck Breast (cooked ,stewed or broiled)	100 grams	133	26.22	0	2.38	0
Duck Leg (cooked ,stewed or broiled)	100 grams	178	29.1	0	5.96	0
Turkey breast (cooked , stewed or broiled)	100 grams	135	30	0	0.74	0
Turkey thighs (cooked , stewed or broiled)	101 grams	196	17	0	13.4	0
Turkey wings (cooked , stewed or broiled)	102 grams	227	27	0	12	0

Food Name	Qty	Cals.	Protein	Carb	Fats	Fibers
Rabbit Meat Cooked Roasted	100 grams	197	29	0	8	0
Americana Beef Shawerma	100 grams	185	24.5	3.2	8.55	2.8
Americana Chicken Shawerma	100 grams	192	16	5	12	0
Eggs Whole	100 grams	147	12.58	0.77	9.94	0
Egg Whites	100 grams	52	10	0.7	0.2	0
Eggology Egg Whites	100 grams	52.156	10.608	0.884	0	0
Luncheon	100 grams	216	18	4	14	0
Pepperoni	100 grams	494	23	0	44	0
Pastrami	100 grams	105	22.7	0.2	1.5	0
Lamb liver raw	100 grams	139	20	1.8	5	0
Beef Liver (cooked ,stewed or broiled)	100 grams	191	29	5	5	0
Chicken Liver (cooked ,stewed or broiled)	100 grams	167	24.5	1	6.5	0
Chicken Heart (cooked ,stewed or broiled)	100 grams	185	26.5	0	7.9	0

Food Name	Qty	Cals.	Protein	Carb	Fats	Fibers
Chicken Gizzared Cooked	100 grams	154	30.1	0	2.7	0
Salami	100 grams	336	22	1	26	0
Tuna Canned in Oil Drained	100 grams	198	29	0	8	0
Tuna canned in oil undrained	100 grams	290	20.8	0	23.2	0
Tuna Canned in Water Drained	100 grams	116	26	0	1	0
Goody Light meat Tuna Sunflower Oil	100 grams	207	28.3	0	10.4	0
John West Tuna drained	100 grams	180	27	0	8	0
Tuna rio marie olive oil	100 grams	360	18	0	32	0
John West Spreadables Tuna Mediterranean	100 grams	184	13	5.5	12	0
Canned Anchovy Drained	100 grams	210	28.89	0	9.71	0
Canned Salmon Drained	100 grams	144	20.5	0	6.28	0

Food Name	Qty	Cals.	Protein	Carb	Fats	Fibers
Carrefour canned salmon	100 grams	170	20	1.7	10	0
Nile Perch Fish Raw	100 grams	82	17	2	0	
Basa fillet cooked	100 grams	107	21	0	1	0
Gilt-Head bream cooked	100 grams	88	20	0	1	0
Mullet Fish (cooked ,stewed or broiled)	100 grams	150	24.81	0	4.86	0
Tilapia Fish (cooked ,stewed or broiled)	100 grams	128	26	0	3	0
Salmon (cooked ,stewed or broiled)	100 grams	171	24	0.49	7.56	0
Parrot Fish cooked	100 grams	150	28	0	2	
Seabream cooked	100 grams	77	17	0	1	0
Russian Zander Fish	100 grams	84	18	0	1	0
Shrimps (cooked ,stewed or broiled)	100 grams	154	24.47	1.17	5.03	0
Supreme Fish cooked	100 grams	88	16	4	1	0

Food Name	Qty	Cals.	Protein	Carb	Fats	Fibers
Red Emperor Fish Raw	100 grams	110	20	0	1	0
Fish Carp cooked dry heat	100 grams	162	23	0	7	0
Grouper Fish Raw	100 grams	92	19	0	1	0
Grouper fish cooked dry heat	100 grams	118	25	0	1	0
Squid (cooked ,stewed or broiled)	100 grams	105	17.9	3.5	1.6	0
Spanish Mackerel cooked dry heat	100 grams	158	24	0	6	0
Mackerel Atlantic Raw	100 grams	205	18.6	0	13.9	0
Crab (raw)	100 grams	86	17	59	1	0
Lizard Fish Cooked	100 grams	93	20.1	0	0.8	0
Red Bream fish	100 grams	143	23	1	5	0
Fish, herring, Atlantic, pickled	100 grams	262	14	3	18	0
Sea Bass Cooked Broiled	100 grams	148	22.1	0.5	5.8	0
Canned Sardines with bones	100 grams	208	24	0	12	0

Food Name	Qty	Cals.	Protein	Carb	Fats	Fibers
Sardine canned in oil undrained	100 grams	298	19	0	25	0
Sardine Whole cooked	100 grams	199	24	0	11	0
Morrison Sardines with Tomato Sauce	100 grams	139	17	1	7	0
Caviar	100 grams	264	25	4	18	0
Greek yogurt	100 grams	87	7	13	3	0
Low Fat Greek Yogurt	100 grams	59	11	4	1	0
Milk Full Cream	100 grams	60	3	5	3	0
Milk Reduced Fat	100 grams	50	3.3	4.68	1.97	0
Milk Skimmed	100 grams	35	3	5	0.2	0
Al-Ain reduced fat milk	100 grams	44	3.2	4.8	3	0
Joya flavoured soya milk Vanilla	100 grams	60	3	8	2	0.5
Camel Milk Full cream	100 grams	46	3	5	2	0
Almond Milk Fortified	100 grams	25	0.4	3.3	1	0.4
Sweet condensed milk	100 grams	325	6.9	56.4	8	0

Food Name	Qty	Cals.	Protein	Carb	Fats	Fibers
Condensed milk unsweetened	100 grams	144	6.9	11	8	0
Arla Protein yogurt	100 grams	62	4.1	9.7	0.5	0
Roamy Cheese	100 grams	374	25	1	30	0
Cheddar Cheese	100 grams	403	24.9	1.28	33.14	0
Edam Cheese	100 grams	356	25	1.4	28	0
Marai Cheddar Cheese Slices	100 grams	270	15	3	22	0
Low Fat Cheddar Cheese	100 grams	173	24.9	1.91	7	0
Low Fat Cheddar Cheese	100 grams	257	19	2	19	0
Cheese Slices Fat free	100 grams	145	21	9	1.5	0
Mersin White Cheese	100 grams	225	5	3	20	0
Turkish Labneh Lite	100 grams	173	8.2	7	12.5	0
Hungarian Cheese	100 grams	210	9	3	18	0
Ricotta cheese	100 grams	174	11	3	13	0

Food Name	Qty	Cals.	Protein	Carb	Fats	Fibers
Frico Edam light	100 grams	317	26	0	24	0
Feta Cheese	100 grams	264	14.21	4.09	21.28	0
Low Fat Feta Cheese	100 grams	176	15.1	2.5	13.1	0
Low fat feta cheese	100 grams	184	14.5	5.3	11.6	0
Domy Feta light	100 grams	150	15.708	5.712	11.424	0
Cottage Cheese	100 grams	103	12.49	2.68	4.51	0
Light Cottage Cheese	100 grams	60	11	3	1	0
Cream Cheese	100 grams	349	7.55	2.66	34.87	0
Light Cream Cheese	100 grams	188	9.4	6.3	14.1	0
Mozzarell a Full Cream	100 grams	318	21.6	2.47	24.64	0
Mozzarell a low Fat	100 grams	254	24.26	2.77	15.92	0
Halloumi Full Cream	100 grams	316	20	1.6	24.7	0
Halloumi Low Fat	100 grams	253	24	3	16	0
Halloumi Low Fat	100 grams	253	23	2	17	0
Low fat Cheddar spread	100 grams	260	11.5	5	21.5	0
Puck low fat white cheese	100 grams	160	15	5	8	0

Food Name	Qty	Cals.	Protein	Carb	Fats	Fibers
Philadelphia light soft cheese	100 grams	128	6.6	5	8.8	0.4
Labneh Diet	100 grams	62	11	1.2	1.5	0
Pinar traditional white cheese	100 grams	260	14	4	21	0
Bahcivan white cheese	100 grams	298	15	1	26	0
Buttermilk	100 grams	60	3	5	3	0
Milk cream	100 grams	345	2.1	2.8	37	0
Light Cream	100 grams	195	2.7	3.66	19.31	0
Yogurt Full cream	100 grams	95	2.9	13	2.7	0
Yogurt Reduced fat	100 grams	63	5	7	2	0
Yogurt Low Fat	100 grams	57	4.6	7	1.1	1
Yoghurt Skim Milk	100 grams	44	5.6	6.3	0.3	0
Vital fresh milk	100 grams	50	3.1	4.8	1.4	0
Yoplait Yogurt Mixed Berries Low Fat	100 grams	91.6	4.1	16.8	0.9	0.3
Chocolate Pudding	100 grams	140	2.1	23	4.6	0
Fage yogurt 2% fat	100 grams	75	10	4	2	0

Food Name	Qty	Cals.	Protein	Carb	Fats	Fibers
Icecream	100 grams	207	3.5	21	11	0.7
Cheesecake	100 grams	321	6	26	1.6	0.4
Kunafa	100 grams	382	1	69	8	8
Pizza	100 grams	209	9.8	24	8.5	2
Jam	100 grams	278	0.4	69	0.1	1.1
Light Jam	100 grams	160	0	32	0	0
Deemah Rich oats biscuits	100 grams	466	10	66.66	20	3.33
Nutella	100 grams	520	7.3	10.7	7.3	0
Jelly	100 grams	278	0.4	67.8	0.1	0
Custard	100 grams	242	6.1	35.6	8.3	0
Cinabbon Classic	100 grams	380	5	54	17	1
Serious Mass	100 grams	375	15	84	1	1
Muscle-Tech Phase 8	100 grams	380	62	19	3.57	
Chike High protein coffee	100 grams	420	60	27	7.5	0
Whey Protein	100 grams	336	75	9	0	0
Myprotein Iso 97	100 grams	399	97	0	1	0.8
Casein Protein	100 grams	336	75	9	0	0
Dymatize Iso 100	100 grams	375	78.126	6.25	1.56	1

Food Name	Qty	Cals.	Protein	Carb	Fats	Fibers
Dymatize Elite Casein	100 grams	393.9399	75.7575	9.09099	0	0
Isopure Zero Carb	100 grams	344.4	82	0	1.64	0
NOW Vanilla Whey Protein	100 grams	395	60.4	16.27	4.65	4.65
NOW Strawberry Whey Protein	100 grams	375	78.125	6.25	1.5625	3.125
Mars Whey Protein	100 grams	386	67.5	11.4	7.3	0
Milk Protein Concentrate	100 grams	365	70	18	1.5	0
Whole milk powder	100 grams	495	26	38	17	0
Dano powder light	100 grams	405	28	48	11	0
Flapjacked Protein pancake and baking mix	100 grams	377.35	37.73	43.39	6.6	9.43
Regilait Powdered Skimmed milk	100 grams	356	35.5	51.7	0.8	1
Protein Bar	100 grams	416	42	17	23	7
Pure protein bar	100 grams	360	40.1	34	9	4

Food Name	Qty	Cals.	Protein	Carb	Fats	Fibers
Detour protein bar chocolate chip	100 grams	397	35.1	39.78	10.53	2.34
Lift low carb protein bar	100 grams	363	34	6.7	13	17
Barebells Cookies and Cream Protein Bar	100 grams	358	36	30	12	6.1
Dymatize Elite Protein Bar	100 grams	383.4	40	34.272	9.996	5.71
Mars Protein	100 grams	351	33	39	8.1	0
Snicker's Protein	100 grams	391	36	36.1	5.3	0
Nestle Fitness Chocolate	100 grams	395	8	74	6	6
Arrowwheat Mills organic buckwheat	100 grams	355	11	69	11.111	
Quest Protein Bar S'mores	100 grams	328	33.33	36.66	14.9999	21.666
Quest Protein bar cookies and cream	100 grams	349.99	35	33.333	14.999	21.666
Max sport protein bar	100 grams	361	25	32.4	14	

Food Name	Qty	Cals.	Protein	Carb	Fats	Fibers
Think Thin High protein bar White chocolate	100 grams	383.33	33.33333	39.99999	13.33333	0
Yogurt Skim Milk	100 grams	56	5.73	7.68	0.18	0
Oats raw	100 grams	347	14	57	7	10
100% Wholegrain Oats	100 grams	375	12.5	67.5	7.5	10
Granola	100 grams	443	12	54	22	8
Fitness Granola Oats Pumkin Seeds Cranberry	100 grams	411	10	67	10	6.7
Nestle Fitness Fruits	100 grams	363	7.4	73.8	2.7	6.9
Weetabix Protein crunch	100 grams	379	20	66	2.5	6.1
Weetabix 100% Whole Grain	100 grams	362	12	69	2	10
Nature Valley Oats and Chocolate	100 grams	456	8.33	60	20	7.14
Museli dried fruit and nuts	100 grams	340	9.7	77.8	4.9	7.3
Fava Beans cooked , boiled	100 grams	110	7.6	19.7	0.4	5.4

Food Name	Qty	Cals.	Protein	Carb	Fats	Fibers
California Fava Beans Egyptian Recipe	100 grams	123	5.383	12.3	5.3	5.3
California Garden Peeled Fave beans	100 grams	100	5.383	9.228	4.614	3.076
Raw Fava Beans	100 grams	341	26	58	2	25
White Rice Raw	100 grams	358	6	79	1	3
Raw Basmati Rice	100 grams	356	6.7	80	1.1	1
White Rice (cooked ,boiled)	100 grams	129	2.66	27.9	0.28	0.4
Brown Rice (cooked ,boiled)	100 grams	112	2.32	23.51	0.83	1.8
Basmati Rice (cooked ,boiled)	100 grams	120.00	3.52	25.08	0.38	0.4
Rice Cakes	100 grams	386.00	8	82	2.8	4.2
Biona Organic rice cakes with quinoa	100 grams	389.00	9.1	78	3.6	3.8
Asian Oreintal Nuts mix	100 grams	506.00	17	52	26	13
Instant Noodles	100 grams	138.00	4.5	2.1	1.2	

Food Name	Qty	Cals.	Protein	Carb	Fats	Fibers
Black eyed peas raw	100 grams	90	3	19	0.4	5
Cowpea	100 grams	116	8	21	0.5	7
Kidney beans canned drained	100 grams	84	5	16	0	5
White Beans canned drained	100 grams	114	7	21	0	5
Soybeans cooked boiled	100 grams	173	17	10	9	6
Chick Peas	100 grams	364	19	61	6	17
Boiled Chickpeas	100 grams	164	8.9	27.42	2.6	8
Canned Chickpeas	100 grams	119	17.2	22.6	9.5	4.4
Lentils	100 grams	353	26	60	1	30
Cooked Lentils	100 grams	116	9	20	0	8
Maggi Corrainder and Garlic mix	100 grams	260	7.7	55	2	2
Lupin	100 grams	120	16	10	3	3
Pasta (cooked ,boiled)	100 grams	158	6	31	1	2
Pasta raw	100 grams	371	13	75	2	3
Whole wheat spaghetti raw	100 grams	352	11.5	67	2.4	12

Food Name	Qty	Cals.	Protein	Carb	Fats	Fibers
Luisine Sliced Brown bread	100 grams	233	9.8	40.1	2.5	5.6
Sliced bran bread	100 grams	234	12.8	33	2.5	13
Luisine brown bread sandwich roll	100 grams	263.9	10.4	46.4	2.8	5.2
Luisine square	100 grams	278	11.19	44.7	4.76	5.6
Multi Cereal bread	100 grams	242	11	37	5	5
Modern Bakery Protein bread	100 grams	266	27.9	7.9	11.1	5.6
whole Wheat flour	100 grams	339	14	73	2	12
Whole Wheat Bread	100 grams	266	9	55	2.6	7.4
Rice bread	100 grams	243	9	44	4.6	4.9
X-Tra fiber Wooden Bakery	100 grams	290	11.4	58	1.4	8
Wholemeal bread	100 grams	235	8.1	44	2.95	3.2
banana bread	100 grams	326	4	55	11	1
Rusk sticks	100 grams	408	12	69.7	7.3	2.8
Rye Crispbread	100 grams	366	8	82	1.3	16

Food Name	Qty	Cals.	Protein	Carb	Fats	Fibers
White bread	100 grams	275	9.1	55.7	2.2	2.4
High Protein Pita	100 grams	216	18.3333	38.3333	1.6888	5.16
French Bread (Vienna, Sourdough)	100 grams	289	11.2	56.4	1.8	2.4
Barley Bread	100 grams	282	8.46	54.7	3.3	5.7
Rye Rusks	100 grams	374	11	70	4.2	8
Psyllium Husk	100 grams	378	0	89	0	78
Croissant	100 grams	406	8	46	21	2.6
White Flour	100 grams	364	10	76	1	2.7
Wheat durum	100 grams	339	14	71	2.5	14
Bread Crumbs	100 grams	395	13.35	71.98	5.3	4.5
Bulgur Cooked	100 grams	83	3.1	18.6	0.2	4.5
Quinoa Cooked	100 grams	120	4.4	21.3	1.9	2.8
Couscous cooked	100 grams	112	3.8	23.2	0.2	1.4
Sweet Potato cooked	100 grams	76	1.37	17.72	0.14	2.5
Boiled Potato	100 grams	103	1.81	19.52	2.24	1.7
Grilled Potato	100 grams	149	2.3	20.1	7	2.5
Potato Chips	100 grams	547	6.56	49.74	37.47	4.4

Food Name	Qty	Cals.	Protein	Carb	Fats	Fibers
Protein Bites Chips	100 grams	387	50	30	6.5	5.3
Fried Potato	100 grams	340	4	44	16	4
Ketchup	100 grams	97	1.7	25.08	0.38	0.3
Tomato Paste	100 grams	82	4	19	0	4
Regular Mayonnaise	100 grams	717	1.1	3.9	78.2	0
Light Mayonnaise	100 grams	324	0.88	8.2	33.09	0
Fat free thousand Island	100 grams	67	0	17	0	0
Mustard	100 grams	66	4.4	5	4	3.3
Balsamic Vingear	100 grams	88	0.5	17	0	0
White Sugar	100 grams	389	0	99.6	0	0
Coffee Creamer	100 grams	545	4.8	55	35.5	0
Nescafe 3 in 1	100 grams	462	1.875	82.5	13.125	0
Honey	100 grams	304	0.3	82.4	0	0.2
Molasses	100 grams	289	0	75	0	0
Dates Molasses	100 grams	305	0	73	0	3
Brown Sugar	100 grams	377	0	97.33	0	0
Cocoa Powder	100 grams	227	20	58	14	33
Snicker's Bar	100 grams	473	7	61	24	2.5

Food Name	Qty	Cals.	Protein	Carb	Fats	Fibers
dark chocolate 70%	100 grams	599	8	46	43	11
Dark chocolate 90%	100 grams	592	10	14	55	
Corona Dark Chocolate	100 grams	502	4.8	55.2	29.6	6
Biscuits	100 grams	366	6	49	17	1.5
Mars Bar	100 grams	467	8	62	23	2
Mcvities Digestive Biscuits	100 grams	447	7.3	70	14.4	3.6
Gateux	100 grams	415	5.2	58	18	2
Pancakes	100 grams	227	6.8	28.7	9.3	0
Malt Beverage	100 grams	37	0.21	8.05	0.12	0
Corn dry	100 grams	419	14	67	11	21
Corn Boiled	100 grams	86	3.22	19.02	1.18	2.7
Corn Fire Roasted	100 grams	111	3.3	24.4	1.1	3.3
Cereal	100 grams	376	7.24	83.02	3.38	5.3
Kelloggs Special K	100 grams	375	9	79	1.5	4.5
Kelloggs coco pops	100 grams	381	9	78	2.5	5
Corn Starch	100 grams	381	0.3	91	0.1	1
Olive oil	100 grams	884	0	0	100	0
Corn Oil	100 grams	884	0	0	100	0

Food Name	Qty	Cals.	Protein	Carb	Fats	Fibers
Fish Oil	100 grams	902	0	0	100	0
Sunflower Oil	100 grams	884	0	0	100	0
Butter	100 grams	717	0.85	0.06	81.11	0
Becel light butter	100 grams	336	0	0.5	38	0
Lard	100 grams	900	0	0	0	
Cooking Cream	100 grams	345	2	3	37	0
Pomegranate Molasses	100 grams	180	0	45	0	0
Olives	100 grams	115	0.8	6	11	3.2
Peanuts	100 grams	599	28.03	15.26	52.5	9.4
Mixed nuts	100 grams	615	15.5	17	56.2	5.5
Castani Kri Kri	100 grams	500	16.6666	43.33333	30	3.33333
Pine Nuts	100 grams	673	14	13	68	3.7
flax seeds	100 grams	534	18	29	42	27
chia seed	100 grams	460	16	44	31	38
Pumpkin Seeds	100 grams	446	19	54	19	18
Sunflower seeds	100 grams	584	21	20	51	9
Pistachio	100 grams	557	20.61	27.97	44.44	10.3
Cashew	100 grams	553	18.22	30.19	43.85	3.3
Walnuts	100 grams	654	15.23	13.71	65.21	6.7

Food Name	Qty	Cals.	Protein	Carb	Fats	Fibers
Coconut	100 grams	667	7	27	67	13
Almonds	100 grams	578	21.26	19.74	50.64	11.8
Sesame Seeds	100 grams	572	18	23	50	12
Peanut Butter	100 grams	588	25.09	19.56	50.39	6
Skippy roasted honey peanut butter	100 grams	625	21.87	18.75	50	6.25
Skippy reduced fat peanut butter	100 grams	500	19.444	41.66	33.33	5.5555
Peanut butter and co dark chocolate dreams	100 grams	531.25	18.75	37.5	40.625	6.5
Whole earth smooth organic peanut butter	100 grams	643	27.7	7.4	54.3	6.7
Pistachio Butter	100 grams	534	19	32	41	10
Tahini	100 grams	595	17	21	54	9
Halvah	100 grams	533	11	32	44	6
Banana	100 grams	89	1.09	22.84	0.33	2.6
Annona	100 grams	75	1.6	14.7	0.7	3
Orange	100 grams	47	0.94	11.75	0.12	2.4

Food Name	Qty	Cals.	Protein	Carb	Fats	Fibers
Orange Juice	100 grams	45	0.7	10	0.2	0.2
Apple Juice	100 grams	46	0.1	11	0.1	0.2
Floridas Natural Orange Pineapple	100 grams	55	0.5	13	0	0
Pomegranate Juice	100 grams	54.5	0.2	13	0.3	0.1
Apple	100 grams	52	0.26	13.81	0.17	2.4
Grapes	100 grams	69	0.72	18.1	0.16	0.9
Watermelon	100 grams	30	0.61	7.55	0.15	0.4
Honeydew melon	100 grams	36	0.54	9.09	0.14	0.8
Cantaloupe	100 grams	34	0.84	8.16	0.19	0.9
Prickly Pears	100 grams	41	0.7	9.6	0.5	3.6
Fig	100 grams	74	0.8	19.2	0.3	2.9
Papaya	100 grams	42.8	0.5	11	0.3	1.7
Peach	100 grams	39	0.91	9.54	0.25	1.5
Plum	100 grams	46	0.7	11.42	0.28	1.4
Apricot	100 grams	48	1.4	11.12	0.39	2
Avocado	100 grams	160	2	8.53	14.66	6.7
Tangerine	100 grams	53	0.81	13.34	0.31	1.8
Grapefruit	100 grams	32	0.6	8.1	0.1	1.1
Cherries	100 grams	63	1	16	0	2

Food Name	Qty	Cals.	Protein	Carb	Fats	Fibers
Black berries	100 grams	43	1.4	10.2	0.5	5.3
Goji Berries	100 grams	357.1	10.713	75	0	7
Mango	100 grams	65	0.51	17	0.27	1.8
Dates	100 grams	282	2.45	75.03	0.39	8
Persimmon	100 grams	70	0.58	18.6	0.19	3.6
Strawberry	100 grams	32	0.67	7.68	0.3	2
Kiwi	100 grams	61	1.14	14.7	0.52	3
Pomegranate	100 grams	68	0.95	17.17	0.3	0.6
Pineapple	100 grams	48	0.54	12.63	0.12	1.4
Pumpkin Raw	100 grams	26.1	1	7	0.1	0.5
Guava	100 grams	68	2.55	14.32	0.95	5.4
Pears	100 grams	58	0.38	15.46	0.12	3.1
Berries	100 grams	57	1	14	0	2
Fruit Salad	100 grams	50	0.5	13	0	1
Raisins	100 grams	299	3.07	79.18	0.46	3.7
Dried Cranberries	100 grams	308	0.1	82	0.7	6
Dried Blueberries	100 grams	320	2	76	0	6

Food Name	Qty	Cals.	Protein	Carb	Fats	Fibers
Dried Apricot	100 grams	241	3.4	62.6	0.5	7.3
Dried figs	100 grams	249	3.3	64	0.9	10
Qamar Aldeen	100 grams	350	3.4	84	0.4	6
Carob	100 grams	323	5	81	1	7
Tamarind	100 grams	239	2.8	63	0.6	5
Frozen mixed vegetables	100 grams	64	3.33	13.46	0.52	4
Fresh Express Farmer's Garden	100 grams	23.5	1.176	3.529	0	1.176
Cucumbers	100 grams	15	0.65	3.63	0.11	0.5
Tomato	100 grams	18	0.88	3.92	0.2	1.2
Artichoke cooked	100 grams	53	2.9	12	0.3	8.6
Radish	100 grams	15.5	0.7	3.4	0.1	
Parsley	100 grams	36	2.97	6.33	0.79	3.3
Onions	100 grams	40	1.1	9	0.1	1.7
Leeks	100 grams	60	1.5	14	0.3	1.8
Beets	100 grams	43	1.6	10	0.2	2.8
Molokhia – Tossa Jute	100 grams	38	4.8	6.3	0.5	5.9
Frozen Molokhia	100 grams	15.35	0.9	2.46	0.4	2.46
Watercress	100 grams	11	2.3	1.29	0.1	0.5

Food Name	Qty	Cals.	Protein	Carb	Fats	Fibers
Celery	100 grams	14	0.69	2.97	0.17	1.6
Celery Juice	100 grams	18	0.83	4	0.16	1.6
Taro	100 grams	112.1	1.5	26	0.2	4.1
Cabbage	100 grams	24	1.44	5.58	0.12	2.3
Broccoli	100 grams	34	2.82	6.64	0.37	2.6
Dill	100 grams	43	3.46	7.02	1.12	2.1
Rosemary	100 grams	131	3.31	20.7	5.86	14.1
Basil	100 grams	27	2.54	4.34	0.61	3.9
Lettuce	100 grams	14	0.9	2.97	0.14	1.2
Carrots	100 grams	41	0.93	9.58	0.24	2.8
Bell Pepper	100 grams	26	0.99	6.03	0.3	2
Mushrooms	100 grams	22	3.09	3.28	0.34	1
Zucchini	100 grams	17	1.2	3.1	0.3	1
Frozen Spinach	100 grams	29	4	4	1	3
Spinach	100 grams	23	2.9	3.6	0.4	2.2
Green Peas	100 grams	81	5	14	0.4	5
Okra	100 grams	33	1.9	7	0.2	3.2
Green Beans	100 grams	31	1.8	7	0.1	3
Eggplant	100 grams	25	1	6	0.2	3
Cauliflower	100 grams	25	1.98	5.3	0.1	2.5

Food Name	Qty	Cals.	Protein	Carb	Fats	Fibers
Garlic	100 grams	148	6	33	0.5	2.1
Unsweetened Iced Tea	100 ml	1	0.01	0.28	0	0
Diet Cola	100 mg	1	0	0	0	0
maple syrup	100 grams	261	0	67	0	0
Lite syrup Chocolate flavor	100 grams	117	0	35	0	0
Subway Chicken Teriyaki 6 inch	100 grams	360	25	57	4.5	5
Chicken spring rolls	100 grams	138	7	14	5	0.8
Americana Chicken Cordon Bleu	100 grams	240	14	19	12	1
Subway Oven Roasted Chicken 6 inch	100 grams	320	23	45	5	5
Subway Chicken Fajita 6 inch	100 grams	340	22	50	7	5
Macdonald's Big Tasty	100 grams	520	27	43	26	4
Macdonald's Quarter Pounder	100 grams	520	30	41	26	3
Hardee's Super Star	100 grams	790	40	41	53	6

Food Name	Qty	Cals.	Protein	Carb	Fats	Fibers
Hardee's Oreo Milk Shake	100 grams	700	14	86	33	1
Macdonald's Mcflory	100 grams	510	12	60	17	2
Halwani Bros Hamburger	100 grams	167.3	13	9.7	8.5	0.3
President Low Fat Cheddar Cheese	100 grams	181.9	17	8	9.1	0
Frico light gouda cheese	100 grams	240	33	0	12	0
President extra light 0.9% fat	100 grams	117	20.5	6.6	0.9	0
Philadephia Cheese Spread Light	100 grams	128	6.6	5	8.8	0.4
President White Lite Cheese	100 grams	131	12	5	7	0
Halwani Bros Minced Meat	100 grams	107.5	17	0	13.5	0
The Three Cows Shredded mozarrella cheese	100 grams	300	22	25	0.8	0
Sliced Coopoliva	100 grams	645	4	0	65	16
Frozen Felafel	100 grams	72.7	3.3	10	1.3	0

Food Name	Qty	Cals.	Protein	Carb	Fats	Fibers
Philadelphia Freekeh	100 grams	59	1.4	13	0.2	0.3
Basak Broccoli cream soup	100 grams	19.6	0.52	3.6	0.32	0.2
Basak Mushroom cream soup	100 grams	81.7	2.2	15	1.2	0.33
Basak Star noodle vegatable soop	100 grams	22.4	0.56	4.48	0.2	0.24
Quaker Vegetables Cumin and Oats Soup	100 grams	51.6	1.84	6.5	1.84	1.2
cheddar cheese Low fat	100 grams	257	19	2	19	0
Tortilla	100 grams	307	9	55	5.35	5
Milk Low fat	100 grams	43.6	3.4	4.9	2	0
Nestle fitness Cereals made with whole grain	100 grams	367	9.67	74.8	1.7	7.5
Chapatti	100 grams	289.55	13.89	48.75	4.25	5
Iko oat bran sugar free	100 grams	510	8	67	13	10
White flour	100 grams	273	11	52	2	3

Food Name	Qty	Cals.	Protein	Carb	Fats	Fibers
All bran flakes Kelloggs	100 grams	359	12	63	3.2	15
Greek Yogurt	100 grams	116	10.2	6.61	5.5	0.96
Mafrood bread	100 grams	275	10	56	1	7
Toast almethaly	100 grams	273	11	52	2	3
Up Salted milk syrup	100 grams	34.6	2.4	3.6	1.1	0
White toast bread square	100 games	256	13	45	2.5	1
Galaxy chocolate Smooth dark	100 grams	520	5.7	59.1	33	14
Granola dark chocolate and red berries love crunch	100 grams	470	6.5	65	19	6.5
Life Protein Icecream	100 grams	153	13.07	15.38	1.923	0
Mozarella low fat	100 grams	235	25	0	15	0
Papaya	100 grams	43	1	11	0	2
Puck Bechamel Sauce with cheese	100 grams	175	5	7	14	0
Craft Cheddar	100 grams	320	20	0	27	0

Food Name	Qty	Cals.	Protein	Carb	Fats	Fibers
Vital Stirred Yogurt Mango and Peach	100 grams	100	3	19.1	1.1	0
Pride Cheese Extra Light	100 grams	117	20.5	6.6	1	0
Pride Cheese Extra Light	100 grams	117	20.5	6.6	1	0
Mcvities Digestive – Dark Chocolate Biscuits	100 grams	495	6	61	24	4
Maxim protein bar	100 grams	356	40	24	12	8
Maltesers	100 grams	500	8.3	61.5	24.3	1.2
Americana Beef Burgers	100 grams	196	15.7	2	13.4	1
pofak kuwait	100 grams	530	7.17	58	32	1.1
Protein bar Barebells caramel &cashew	100 grams	361	36	26	15	7.9
Chechil cheese	100 grams	322	25	1.6	24	0
Luisine cream cheese sandwich	100 grams	303	9.7	36	13	1.6
Greek yogurt blueberry	100 grams	94	5	14	2	0

Food Name	Qty	Cals.	Protein	Carb	Fats	Fibers
Yogurt strawberries	100 grams	105	4	15.5	3	0
Jelly Cranberry Greens	100 grams	61	1.79	13.7	0.4	0
Luna Red kidney beans	100 grams	149	9.8	20	0.2	7
Cooked Mackerel	100 grams	222	22.5	0.4	13.8	0
Skimmed milk Almarai	100 grams	33.8	3.2	5	0.1	0
Cream Light Almarai	100 grams	166	3.3	4.4	15	0
Bechamel sauce with cheese Puck	100 grams	117	20.5	6.6	0.9	0
cheese spread light Philadelphia	100 grams	128	6.6	5	8.8	0.4
Salmon raw	100 grams	131	23	0	4.5	0
Tang orange	100 grams	358	1.4	68	0.1	0.1
Cheese Slices fat free	100 grams	569	21	9	1.5	0
Beef sheesh kebab freshly foods	100 grams	176	23	25	5	2

Food Name	Qty	Cals.	Protein	Carb	Fats	Fibers
Goody Peanut butter low fat	100 grams	450	24.5	32	37	6.5
Impact Whey Isolate Myprotein	100 grams	373	90	2.5	0.3	0
Super Mass Gainer Dymatize	100 grams	381	15.47	72	2.97	1.19
Cooking cream light	100 grams	134	2.6	5.8	12	0
Tuna salad mayonnaise fisherman	100 grams	158	7.7	5.6	11	0
Tanour healthy bread with black seeds	100 grams	400	10	70	0	5
Doline Posni	100 grams	73.5	12	3	1.5	0
Classic White Cheese	100 grams	268	19	0.7	21	0.5
Multi power 100% pure whey	100 grams	379	78	4.3	4.7	1.9
Raw shelled shrimp	100 grams	144	27.5	1.24	2.35	0
Sports Factory Protein Shake 90	100 grams	350	80	4.2	0.9	1.8

Summary of the dieting table of ketogenic :A healthy ketogenic diet should consist of approximately 75% fat, 20% protein and 5% carbohydrates or less than 50 grams of carbohydrates per day.

Focus on high-fat and low-carb foods such as eggs, meat, dairy products and low-carb vegetables, as well as sugar-free drinks. Make sure to restrict unhealthy high-fat processed ingredients. The ketogenic diet is more popular and easier than ever, and you can find a wide range of healthy and interesting ideas online

www.ingramcontent.com/pod-product-compliance
Lightning Source LLC
Chambersburg PA
CBHW040228240726
48664CB00001B/58